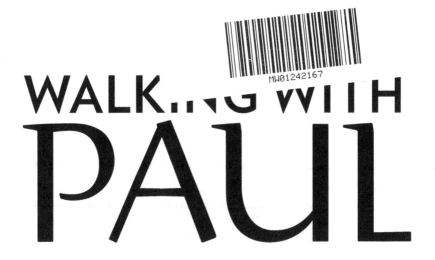

WALKING WITH PAUL

Six weeks of devotions
for body and spirit

Susan Martins Miller

Healthy Living
for Church and Home
✚RESOURCES FROM CHURCH HEALTH

Founded in 1987, Church Health is a charitably funded, faith-based, not-for-profit organization with a mission to *reclaim the church's biblical commitment to care for our bodies and our spirits.* Church Health provides comprehensive, high-quality, affordable health care to uninsured and underserved individuals and their families and gives people tools to live healthier lives. With the generous support of volunteer providers, the faith community, donors and community partners, we work tirelessly to improve health and well-being so that people can experience the full richness of life. For more information visit www.ChurchHealth.org.

Walking with Paul: Six Weeks of Devotions for Body and Spirit
© 2013, 2020 Church Health Center, Inc. Memphis, TN

Scripture quotations contained herein are from the New Revised Standard Version Bible, copyright 1989, Division of Christian Education of the National Council of the Churches of Christ in the United States of America, and are used by permission. All rights reserved.

ISBN: 978-1-62144-067-3

Healthy Living for Church and Home brings you practical tools and insights to help you faithfully create habits to honor God and know fullness of life.

Walking with Paul is part of the Ways to Wellness series, which also includes *Walking with Jesus* and *Walking with Abraham and Sarah.*

Written by Susan Martins Miller.

Cover and interior design by Lizy Heard.

Our Mission

CHURCH HEALTH is a faith-based organization. Each day, we stand ready to care for people who are hurting but live within a health care system that has left them behind. Our neighbors come seeking help, yet what they find is much deeper and more healing. They discover hope for a better life.

The Bible calls us to follow Jesus, which means helping people farther along the path to knowing God by showing God's love through our actions to heal both body and spirit. Because the Bible guides our understanding of God's love as well as God's calling for us, we share the Bible's commitment to bring wellness and hope to people of all circumstances.

We know from history that Christians have always cared for the underserved, both in body and spirit. Jesus asks us to care about what he cares about—wellness and wholeness of all people. Healing that flows through personal care, preventive activities, medical methods, and health technology announce that God is present among us.

God invites us to participate in the overarching story of God's love in the world. The commitment to care for bodies and spirits belongs to the church—both locally and worldwide—because the church belongs to Jesus.

In Memphis, Tennessee, Church Health provides clinical services to uninsured and underserved individuals in the areas of medical, dental, optometry, physical rehabilitation, and behavioral health, along with wellness services in nutrition, life health coaching, child well-being, and disease prevention. Our funding comes from charitable sources, and hundreds of volunteers augment our staff to care for thousands of patients. Beyond Memphis, we reach across the country and around the globe with a ministry of faith community nurses and publications for healthy living.

Your purchase and use of this publication shares in our mission to care for bodies and spirits in a way that shows the love and hope of Jesus on the road to living in healthier ways that honor God's love for us.

For more information visit www.ChurchHealth.org.

Introduction

WELCOME TO *Walking with Paul*, a six-week experience designed to help you make small changes and simple lifestyle improvements in your health and to grow in faith by accomplishing three simple goals:

1. Add 2,000 more steps a day to your activity level.
2. Add 3 servings of vegetables to your daily meals.
3. Add 3 glasses of water (a total of 24 ounces) each day to your daily fluids.

An inspiring devotional dimension reminds you of the connection between health in body and spirit. As you work on physical health goals, daily Scripture readings and meditations help you follow the routes that Jesus walked and nurture your spirit as well.

GETTING STARTED

You may choose to complete *Walking with Paul* on your own, with a friend or two, or as part of a program organized through your congregation or community group.

To get started, you'll want to know the baseline for how many steps you take in a typical day, how many servings of vegetables you eat, and how much water you drink.

1. **STEPS.** If you don't have a good idea of the number of steps you take in a day, plan on using the first three days to maintain a normal activity level, but keep track of your steps. You can use a pedometer or convert minutes of activity into steps using the Activity Conversion Chart on page 11. Average your number of steps during the first three days to set your baseline.

For instance, Tom walked, 5,050 steps on Monday, 4,123 steps on Tuesday, and 6,233 steps on Wednesday. This adds up to a total of 15,406 steps. He'll divide the number by three to get an average of 5,135 steps per day. This is Tom's baseline.

Then the goal will be to increase the daily steps by 2,000. If your baseline is about 5,000 steps, then you'll aim for 7,000 steps each day. If your baseline is 3,000 steps, then you'll aim for 5,000. You won't be comparing yourself to anyone else—only where you've been and where you want to go.

2. **VEGETABLES.** For three days, record how many servings of vegetables you eat. One serving is one-half cup cooked or one cup raw vegetables. Find

your average for the three days. That is your baseline. The goal is to add three more. If your average is two servings, aim for five. If your average is four, aim for seven.

3. **WATER.** For three days, keep track of how many times you drink at least eight ounces of water. Find your average for the three days. That is your baseline. Adding three glasses per day (a total of 24 ounces) can be as simple as drinking eight ounces (one cup) of water at each of three meals.

— MY PERSONAL RECORD —

Program Start Date: ....

My baseline steps ....   My steps goal ....

My baseline vegetables ....   My vegetables goal ....

My baseline water ....   My water goal ....

BENEFITS OF *WALKING WITH PAUL*

The eating and physical activity patterns of the majority of Americans have made us the most overweight nation in the world. More than 60 percent of American adults do not get the recommended 30 minutes of physical activity in a day, and 25 percent are not physically active at all. Nearly two-thirds of adults are overweight, with the average person gaining one or two pounds each year.

This six-week experience will:

- Inspire individuals, groups of friends, or whole congregations to engage in fun, simple ways to become more active and eat more healthfully (and move toward a healthy weight as needed).
- Create a supportive network for changes in individual and congregational behavior.
- Encourage everyone who participates to use their gifts to live a healthy life.

It's all about energy balance! We can manage weight gain by creating a healthier balance between the amount of energy burned and the types and amount of food consumed throughout a normal day. Small changes, such as the three goals in this program, can make a difference without creating a sense of impossibility or failure. The key is reasonable and achievable goals. Big change doesn't happen all at once, but one step at a time—literally.

TOOLS IN THIS BOOK

You'll want to keep a Bible handy as you read each day's meditation. Many Bibles include maps that may help you identify locations mentioned in the passages you read. A simple **MAP**, such as on the back cover, gives you an appreciation for the places and distances Jesus traveled.

Each day's reading page also includes a **DAILY HEALTH JOURNAL** where you can record your number of steps for that day and check off whether you met the goals of adding 2,000 steps, 3 servings of vegetables, and 3 glasses of water. At the end of each week, transfer your checkmarks to a summary chart and see how you did for the week overall.

In addition to the daily meditations, each day provides a new **HEALTH TIP** to share health information or encourage you to incorporate what you already know into your daily routines.

At the close of this introductory material, you'll also find **TIPS FOR ADDING STEPS TO YOUR DAY** and an **ACTIVITY CONVERSION CHART** to help you calculate how other physical activity equates to added steps. Bicycling, gardening, yoga, rollerblading—it all counts toward walking. If you would also like to trim calories, a bonus goal, you'll find **TIPS FOR CUTTING 100 CALORIES**.

To begin your six weeks of walking, consider using the Self-assessment on page 13 that invites you to record you baseline habits and attitudes. Share this with a friend or turn it in to a project coordinator if you are part of a congregational program. At the end of six weeks, you'll have another opportunity to answer similar questions, evaluate your progress, and set new goals.

WALKING WITH PAUL IN A GROUP

Many features of *Walking with Paul* are for individual use—keeping the Daily Health Journal, setting personal goals, and seeking spiritual inspiration in the daily reflections you can read at any time of the day. This doesn't mean you have to be on your own. You might be a leader looking for a simple program to use in your congregation to encourage healthy habits, or you might be someone who wants to gather a few friends for a shared path for six weeks of accountability as you all set reasonable goals and support each other in reaching them. Whether a handful of friends or a congregation-wide program, *Walking with Paul* works well for group use.

Here are a few tips.

1. **ORDER COPIES IN ADVANCE.** If you're reading this copy of *Walking with Paul* and want to organize a group, make it easy by ordering copies for your group at one time. Make sure everyone has a copy before the start of the six-week period.

2. **HOLD A BRIEF LAUNCH MEETING.** This doesn't have to be long or involved. The purpose is to draw attention to the tools in the book and agree together how you want to use them in your group. This gets everyone on the same page so that as you support each other over the six-week period, everyone speaks the same language. Will you share the pre- and post-assessments? What do you think will be the best ways you'll want to add steps or cut calories from the tips lists provided? How often will you connect with each other?

3. PLAN WAYS TO TOUCH BASE. Knowing how to support each other will be important. Some ideas are:

- Meet for a few minutes during the coffee time or adult Sunday school hour on Sunday mornings and talk about successes and challenges of the week. Share which reflections encouraged you the most. Pray for one another.

- Set up a closed Facebook group and post daily questions for members to respond to about how they're doing on their health journeys. Consider ways to tie questions to the daily reflections or health tips.

- Use a group e-mail, text message, or Messenger process for frequent private contact with words of encouragement, tips, and brief prayers.

- Plan times when members of the group can physically walk together and share their successes and challenges and get some steps in at the same time. The whole group doesn't have to walk together. This could be a time for two to four people to meet up according to schedules or locations.

4. SHARE A CLOSING MEAL. At the end of six weeks, share a healthy meal. Invite participants who shared the walking journey to bring healthy dishes that reflect ways they changed their eating during the six weeks. There might be some recipe swapping!

Each new healthy habit becomes a foundation for the next one. One of the best ways to celebrate progress is to know your starting point and be able to look back after six weeks and see changes. No change for the better is too small to celebrate.

Choose the stairs instead of the elevator.

Park in the back row of the parking lot.

Mow the lawn with a walking mower.

Walk with a friend during your lunch break.

Pace around the house while talking on the phone.

Instead of e-mailing or calling a coworker, walk down the hall and have a face-to-face interaction.

Make several trips and up and down the stairs when doing laundry and household chores.

Pass the drive-thru and walk into the restaurant or bank.

Tour a museum, zoo, or nature preserve.

Volunteer to walk dogs for an animal shelter.

Walk to yard sales to shop for bargains.

Circle around the block once before bringing in the mail.

Walk on short errands, such as a nearby store, post office, or dry cleaners.

Go window shopping at the mall.

Meet a friend for lunch at a restaurant you can walk to.

Play a round of golf but pass on the golf cart.

TIPS FOR CUTTING 100 CALORIES

Small changes in food preparation and portion size can quickly add up and have a dramatic impact on your health. Each one of these options will allow you to trim 100 calories out of your daily intake and meet your daily goal.

Select skim, one percent or two percent milk instead of whole milk.

Use a small glass for juice and a small bowl for cereal.

Use cooking spray in place of butter or margarine.

Put lettuce, tomato, onions, and pickles on your burger or sandwich instead of cheese.

Prepare tuna or chicken salad with fat-free or light mayonnaise.

Select soft corn tortillas instead of hard shell tortillas.

Replace a can of soda with mineral water.

Enjoy your salad without the croutons.

Leave three or four bites on your plate.

Use a fat-free, light, or reduced-fat cheese, sour cream, or salad dressing in place of regular.

Limit meat portions to three or four ounces—the size of a deck of cards.

Steam vegetables rather than frying with butter.

Add 1/4 less cheese to spaghetti and lasagna. Customize the dish with fresh seasonal vegetables.

Bake, broil, or grill chicken instead of frying.

Share one serving of dessert with a friend.

Substitute applesauce for vegetable oil when baking.

Choose 100 percent juice over juice cocktails and fruit punch.

Skip super-sized portions.

Choose a side salad or steamed vegetables instead of fries, pasta, or onion rings.

Dip your fork in salad dressing instead of pouring dressing over the salad.

Cut out one tablespoon of butter or oil from a recipe.

Use two egg whites in place of one whole egg.

ACTIVITY CONVERSION CHART

If you engage in physical activities other than walking, you can convert minutes of activity to steps for credit toward adding 2,000 steps per day to your usual routine.

Activity	Steps per Minute
Aerobics (low-impact)	125
Aerobics (moderate)	153
Aerobics (water)	100
Basketball	100
Bicycling (leisurely)	100
Bicycling (moderate)	200
Bicycling (stationary)	181
Cross country skiing	114
Dancing (all types)	133
Elliptical machine	203
Football	133
Gardening	73
Golf (walking)	100
Jogging (12 minutes per mile)	232
Hopping	51
Painting	78
Pilates	92
Racquetball	138
Resistance training	74
Rollerblading	200
Rowing (leisurely)	74
Rowing (moderate)	153
Running (10 minutes per mile)	290
Running (7.5 minutes per mile)	391
Scrubbing floors	92
Soccer	144
Stair climbing (down)	72

Continued on page 12.

Continued from page 11.

Activity	Steps per Minute
Stair climbing (up)	205
Stretching	6
Swimming	200
Tai chi	8
Tennis	200
Volleyball	90
Walking	125
Washing car	72
Waterskiing	136
Weight lifting	100
Yoga	50

— Self-assessment —

If you are using Walking with Paul *as part of a group or congregation, answer these questions before you begin and consider sharing your answers with the project coordinator or friends in your group.*

Name: ....

Congregation or Community Organization: ....
....

1. How many days a week do you engage in some type of mild to moderate physical activity (walking slowly, gardening, housework, window shopping, and so on)? Days per week ....

2. How many days a week do you engage in some type of moderate to vigorous physical activity (brisk walking, running, riding a bike, dancing, playing a sport and so on)? Days per week ....

3. Which answer best describes how you feel about the following?

	I have no plans to	I plan to in the future	I plan to immediately	I have been doing so for *fewer* than six months	I have been doing so for *more* than six months
Increasing physical activity					
Improving nutrition					

4. To what degree do you feel that your physical health and spiritual health are connected?

   ○ Not at all   ○ Quite a bit
   ○ A little bit   ○ Extremely
   ○ Moderately

CUT HERE

Begin Your Journey
Here

Meet Paul

ACTS 7:59-8:3

"Lord, do not hold this sin against them."
—Acts 7:60

THE STORY OF THE apostle Paul begins as a footnote to the story of Stephen. Luke, the author of the book of Acts, describes Stephen as "a man full of faith and the Holy Spirit" (Acts 6:5) and "full of grace and power" (Acts 6:8). He was one of seven individuals chosen to assist the apostles leading the early church by attending to practical needs among the believers. Stephen is the first person outside the original disciples that Luke records as working miracles, and for this he was arrested and stoned.

As people gathered to witness Stephen's execution, they laid their coats at the feet of a young man named Saul (Acts 7:58). While he was being stoned, Stephen knelt and prayed for his enemies: "Lord do not hold this sin against them." Stephen died, and Luke tells us, "And Saul approved of their killing him" (Acts 8:1).

Saul was there among the opposition who had been arguing—unsuccessfully—with Stephen. The bandwagon was headed in only one direction, and Saul was on it. We will soon read about Saul's drastic confrontation demanding a change of heart. His life turned in a new direction. In our pursuit of health and wholeness, we may need to be confronted in a dramatic way. We learn from Saul, who became Paul, that change is possible, even for the least likely candidate. No matter what health challenge you face, changing your health habits is possible with God's help.

HEALTH TIP

Stress contributes to many physical problems, including heart disease, stroke, and obesity. Recognizing the effect of stress helps us to manage it better. Being resilient does not mean that we never feel stressed or face adverse conditions, but if we work on healthy habits when we are not stressed, they will serve us well when the tough times come. In small steps, we can move from less satisfying ways of thinking to more positive thoughts and behaviors.

— DAILY HEALTH JOURNAL —

Number of steps............................   O Add 3 servings of vegetables
O Add 2,000 steps   O Add 3 glasses of water

The Light Goes On

ACTS 9:1–5

He asked, "Who are you, Lord?" The reply came,
"I am Jesus, whom you are persecuting."
—Acts 9:5

AFTER STEPHEN'S DEATH, persecution broke out against the first Christians in Jerusalem, and many believers scattered—carrying the good news of Jesus with them. Saul was determined to stamp out this uprising, and the Jewish high priest was more than happy to give him all the authority he needed to find people who believed in Jesus and bring them back to Jerusalem. This is what Saul was doing, on his way to Damascus, when light flashed around him and a voice spoke.

"Who are you?" Saul asked. Put yourself in his place. What could possibly be happening? And the answer came that the voice speaking to Saul was Jesus!

Saul thought he knew everything there was to know about the God he worshipped. He was certain that this man Jesus who had been crucified had nothing to do with true religion or true belief. He was so sure that he was willing to see anyone who believed in Jesus put to death. And this same Jesus stopped Saul in his tracks.

Saul's core belief was challenged. The premise upon which his life was built was proven to be wrong. Jesus had indeed come from God. Because his own experience persuaded him to change what he believed, the door opened for a complete change in the direction of Saul's life.

What belief about yourself, or about how God feels about you, do you need to let go of so that your life can turn toward greater wholeness?

HEALTH TIP

Not everyone's journey toward wellness is identical. Don't try to squeeze your path into someone else's shape. Look through the lens of your own life and what goals are realistic. Even more, consider your personal reasons for wanting to make changes in your well-being. What matters most to you? No two people will answer that question the same way, but it is the essential question in wellness.

— DAILY HEALTH JOURNAL —

Number of steps ....   O Add 3 servings of vegetables

O Add 2,000 steps   O Add 3 glasses of water

Chosen

ACTS 9:10-19

But the Lord came to him, "Go, for he is an instrument
whom I have chosen to bring my name before Gentiles."
—Acts 9:15

THOUGH THE EYES OF HIS HEART were opened, Saul left his encounter with Jesus on the road to Damascus unable to physically see. God was already at work in the next phase of Saul's journey to new faith. In Damascus was a man named Ananias. God spoke to Ananias and told him to go find Saul. Saul's reputation was widely known. Ananias knew how dangerous Saul was to those who believed in Jesus. Should Ananias really walk straight into the face of evil? This instruction from God made no sense.

Luke does not record a long speech of explanation by God to put Ananias at ease, but he does give us God's grand plan: "Go, for he is an instrument whom I have chosen to bring my name before Gentiles." What God asked of Ananias was unexpected. And God's choice of Saul to be an instrument of the gospel, and fulfillment of Old Testament promises of God's care for all people dating back to God's covenant with Abraham recorded in the book of Genesis, must have been mind-boggling to Ananias.

Both Paul and Ananias took risks as they moved toward one another, but both acted in obedience to God. What work, in whatever form we answer the call of God on our lives, is outside your own plan and understanding?

HEALTH TIP

What is your personal attitude toward wellness goals? If you've already decided that "nothing works," change will be difficult. On the other hand, if you're confident that you can make one small change at a time, and develop patience with yourself when you face setbacks, you're more likely to see the results you desire. The journey to wellness is not always easy, but with a positive attitude, the path can smooth out.

— **DAILY HEALTH JOURNAL** —

Number of steps............................   ○ Add 3 servings of vegetables
○ Add 2,000 steps   ○ Add 3 glasses of water

Hard to Believe

ACTS 9:19-25

For several days he was with the disciples in Damascus,
and immediately he began to proclaim Jesus in the synagogues.
—Acts 9:19-20

SAUL WASTED NO TIME IN Damascus. He was baptized and joined the believers in that city. He even began speaking about Jesus in the Jewish synagogues. This was a great reversal of his previous habits! He preached that Jesus was the Son of God, the very claim that had made him so eager to stamp out the rapidly growing Christian movement. The intellect and determination that were part of Saul's personality did not disappear. Instead, his gifts turned to his new calling.

Imagine Ananias baptizing Saul and introducing him to the other believers. Imagine hearing Saul tell the story of meeting Jesus on the road to Damascus. Would you have believed him? Could a person change from night to day so completely? Was it a trick to infiltrate? Would he quickly turn back to his old ways?

On our own journeys, or in seeing the change in others along the wellness road, we might be just as suspicious about whether change is genuine and lasting. Even when we are successful at changing health habits, others might still think of us as the person with our old ways. After all, how many people make resolutions to "get healthy" and fall off the wagon at the first sight of a brownie?

It's easy to fall into the rut of believing real change is not possible. But Saul's story of new belief and new behaviors tells us that change *is* possible.

HEALTH TIP

Hypertension is a disease that develops over time. Heredity plays a role, but so does lifestyle—our choices, behaviors, and habits. Everyday choices may be the results of deeply ingrained habits—so deep that we don't recognize them. But habits are not by definition bad. Now is a good time to make a list of the health-supporting habits you already have and consider how you can build on that foundation.

--- **DAILY HEALTH JOURNAL** ---

Number of steps............................

O Add 2,000 steps

O Add 3 servings of vegetables

O Add 3 glasses of water

Fear of Change

ACTS 9:26-31

But Barnabas took him, brought him to the apostles, and described for them how on the road he had seen the Lord, who had spoken to him.

—Acts 9:27

IN DAMASCUS THE BELIEVERS had the chance to see for themselves the change in Saul. They were so convinced of his genuine change that when Jewish leaders threatened Saul's life, the believers helped him escape (Acts 9:23–24). After a period of time, Saul traveled back to Jerusalem to join the believers. Remember, Jerusalem is where Stephen was stoned and Saul approved of the event. It's the place where persecution of believers broke out on a large scale, and many of the apostles scattered. Can we blame the believers for a fearful response to Saul's return? Some time has passed, and word of Saul's new belief likely had filtered back to Jerusalem. But hearing the story and seeing the person are two different things.

Barnabas was first mentioned in Acts 4:36 because he sold a field and gave the money to leaders of the early church to help take care of the poor. Now Barnabas is the one who steps up to defend Saul and persuade the others to accept him.

Sometimes it takes only one other person to believe along with you that you can make genuine and lasting changes to your health, whether it's weight management, relational wellness, or a needed job change. Maybe you can think of who that person is for you. Let's take our cue from Barnabas and be the person who is an encourager and supporter to others on the health journey.

HEALTH TIP

When people talk about "getting healthier," too often they think that means sweeping changes that take the fun out of life. But drastic all-at-once changes set us up for feeling overwhelmed, failing to stick with our goals, and eventually giving up. Instead, smaller goals that can be sustained over time will make us successful at achieving goals without constantly running into barriers to success. Setting goals that are realistic for *you* is a key step toward improving health.

— DAILY HEALTH JOURNAL —

Number of steps............................ ○ Add 3 servings of vegetables

○ Add 2,000 steps ○ Add 3 glasses of water

Paul's First Journey Begins

ACTS 13:1-5

The Holy Spirit said, "Set apart for me Barnabas
and Saul for the work to which I have called them."
—Acts 13:2

MANY EVENTS HAVE OCCURRED between Acts 9, where Saul was converted and joined the believers, and Acts 13, where his ministry begins in earnest. Writer Luke took some time to tell us what had become of Peter, another giant in the accounts of the early church. Now Luke returns to Saul's story.

Saul and Barnabas have been among the leaders in a church in Antioch. While the believers worshiped, the Holy Spirit spoke to them with instructions to send Barnabas and Saul off with a special calling. Luke stresses that they were appointed by the congregation but also by the Holy Spirit. We see the wisdom of being connected not only to God but to other believers who can help us discern the ways God calls us to serve in our lives and to be partners with us in the ministry we undertake.

When we consider the place that our work has in our overall wellness, we must ponder what place calling has in the obligations we enter into. Not every job will be perfect, but might God call us to that work anyway? Not every job is even paid, such as community committees and other forms of volunteering, but God may shape our spirits by calling us into meaningful experiences.

Have we already decided what we want, or are we listening to how God might surprise us with a new calling by speaking through the people who know us best?

HEALTH TIP

What does it take to change a habit? Habits are the things we do on auto-pilot, the things we reach for without thinking, the familiar movements we do by rote. Habits manifest in food choices, emotional ups and downs, and activity levels. As you go through your day, stop periodically to ask what you've done out of habit. We can change habits that harm our health, and we can reinforce habits that support well-being.

— DAILY HEALTH JOURNAL —

Number of steps............................ ◯ Add 3 servings of vegetables

◯ Add 2,000 steps ◯ Add 3 glasses of water

Staying the Course
ACTS 13:13-16

The officials of the synagogue sent them a message, saying,
"Brothers, if you have any word of exhortation for the people, give it."
—Acts 13:15

BARNABAS AND PAUL—Luke has changed the form he uses of Saul's name—are well into their missionary journey of preaching the good news, teaching in the synagogues, and healing the sick. They arrived in Antioch in Pisidia (a different city than Antioch in Syria, where their journey began). As usual, on the Sabbath they went to the synagogue to worship, and the officials of the synagogue invited them to speak. Paul accepted the opportunity to speak about Jesus.

Throughout the book of Acts, we see that Paul went first to Jewish congregations in synagogues. In some places his message was received positively. In others, he was rejected and even threatened. Either way, we learn the wisdom of waiting for the invitation to speak to others about Jesus and about the role that faith can play in spurring us along on the road to better health.

Perhaps Paul did not know how long this particular missionary journey would last. Perhaps he did not know that he would take several other long missionary journeys. But he knew what the message of his own life would be, and he could wait for God's invitation and timing to speak the words that would affect the lives of many others.

How often are we tempted to blurt out what someone else "should" do or think? Probably too often! Instead, let us sense when God is saying that the time is right to walk alongside others on the path to wellness.

HEALTH TIP

Where is your comfort zone—and how does it affect choices you make about forming healthy habits? Stepping outside your comfort zone and beginning a new journey can stir up anxiety, and a physical reaction begins. Practice taking a few deep, slow breaths in the morning or evening. Then when you face a situation outside your comfort zone, you will know how to slow down, breathe, and remind yourself that you are safe.

— DAILY HEALTH JOURNAL —

Number of steps............................ ○ Add 3 servings of vegetables

○ Add 2,000 steps ○ Add 3 glasses of water

Six weeks of devotions for body and spirit **23**

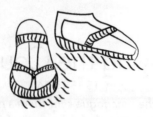

Week One in Review

ARE YOU FINDING LESSONS that resonate as you walk with Paul through the early phases of his ministry? An encounter with Jesus changed his belief and led to turning his life in a direction he had not imagined. He learned from others. He joined with others. He listened to the wisdom of others. He put his God-given abilities to use in the service of others. He was not a lone ranger.

These are lessons we can all take to heart as we take our next steps along the pathway to an improved level of health in all the dimensions of our daily lives—work, relationships, emotions, faith, medical issues, what we eat and how we move. We don't have to do it alone, and as impossible as change might seem, it is possible. The change might not be change in our outward circumstances. It might be better health in our spirits and in our ability to manage the circumstances of our lives in healthier ways.

*Transfer your daily steps in the space below. If you set a goal
for all three categories, put checkmarks in the boxes
where you reached your goal for each day.*

Number of steps	Add 2,000 steps	Add 3 vegetables	Add 3 glasses of water
Day 1	O	O	O
Day 2	O	O	O
Day 3	O	O	O
Day 4	O	O	O
Day 5	O	O	O
Day 6	O	O	O
Day 7	O	O	O

A Message of Good News

ACTS 13:30–33

*"And we bring you the good news that what
God promised to our ancestors he has fulfilled for us."*

—Acts 13:32–33

WE PICK UP AGAIN IN THE middle of the sermon that Paul was giving in the synagogue in Antioch of Pisidia. After reminding his listeners of the ways God had been active on behalf of God's people through the centuries—the beliefs he robustly shared with the hearers—he now turned to speaking boldly about Jesus. His key message was that the salvation that the Hebrew Scriptures spoke of, which God had promised since the time of Abraham, was fulfilled in Jesus.

"We bring you the good news that what God promised to our ancestors he has fulfilled for us," Paul said.

Paul did not force a message upon his listeners without first preparing them by acknowledging where they were on their own spiritual journeys. The power of God, who raised Jesus from the dead, would join them on their journeys. The gospel is God's good news for what God wants for us—what God has wanted for all people from the start.

In lives where bad news can strike at any moment, with the next phone call or the next piece of mail or the next conversation that we have in a typical day, isn't it good news that God's plan has been unwavering? Isn't it good news that God's plan is coming to fulfillment? Isn't it good news that we can participate in God's plan for the world? Take a few minutes to consider how God's good news manifests in your life.

HEALTH TIP

We all run out of energy—and often reach for the wrong foods or don't even want to think about what we're eating. The right foods fuel our bodies, but did you know that socializing with others also revitalizes your energy? People who are often alone and avoid social interaction also report feeling more tired, stressed out, and overwhelmed. Take time to be with friends this week.

— **DAILY HEALTH JOURNAL** —

Number of steps _____   ○ Add 3 servings of vegetables

○ Add 2,000 steps   ○ Add 3 glasses of water

Light for the Gentiles
ACTS 13:44-47

"For so the Lord has commanded us, saying, 'I have set you to be a light for the Gentiles, so that you may bring salvation to the ends of the earth.'"
—Acts 13:47

P AUL AND BARNABAS SPOKE BOLDLY in the synagogue, and people—both Jewish and Gentile—began to follow them. A week later, on the next Sabbath day, a crowd gathered to hear them. Luke describes it as the "whole city." Word of mouth can cover a lot of ground in a week!

Jewish leaders continued to oppose the message Paul and Barnabas preached, but they countered by again quoting Hebrew Scriptures that listeners would have known well. Citing Isaiah 49:6, they emphasized that the prophets had spoken of the coming Messiah—Jesus—as fulfillment of God's promise of salvation. They went further and extended the core message to include those who continue the mission of Jesus. God intended salvation not only for the Jewish people but all people. This is the promise captured in the phrase "a light for the Gentiles."

Paul and Barnabas had a message of good news, and although Jewish leaders opposed them, many in the crowds were eager and receptive. From their boldness in sharing good news, we are challenged to our own boldness with a message of health and healing. First, boldness comes as we demonstrate health in our own pursuit of greater wellness. Then we are also bold in encouraging others to believe that they, too, can experience health in God's care.

HEALTH TIP

Is your life hectic? Most of us would answer yes. Before you plunge into yet another time management strategy in order to "do it all," press pause. What demands on your time and energy are within your ability to control? What brings you joy? What's missing from your life that would bring more joy? What change can you make to be sure your life is not only full of busyness but also full of joy?

--- DAILY HEALTH JOURNAL ---

Number of steps ....

O Add 2,000 steps

O Add 3 servings of vegetables

O Add 3 glasses of water

Rejoicing in Hard Times

ACTS 13:48-52

And the disciples were filled with
joy and with the Holy Spirit.

—Acts 13:52

"**T**HUS THE WORD OF THE LORD** spread throughout the region," Luke tells us (Acts 13:49). With the success Paul and Barnabas had also came opposition. Jewish leaders buckled down to find a strategy to discredit the missionaries. Luke uses a strong word—"incited"—to describe their actions. It was purposeful and meant to cause controversy and public spectacle.

The Jewish leaders called on influential people, both women and men, to do their bidding. Perhaps they called in favors. Perhaps they promised favors. Whatever the reasons that these individuals chose to side with synagogue leaders and others who felt threatened by the message of Jesus, persecution resulted. Public pressure forced Paul and Barnabas out of the area.

Even in our own decisions about health and wellness, we may find ourselves wondering what the influential people think. Does a favorite celebrity espouse a particular way of eating? Do family members try to tell us what we should or should not be doing for exercise or managing stress? What does the pastor think? Do we try one thing and then another because we're not sure? Do our friends seem to disparage our intentions?

All these experiences can pull us away from the central message that God cares about our wellness and that when we care for both body and spirit we honor God. Find the good news not in quick fixes or advice but in hearing God's voice calling you to a life filled with the joy God gives.

HEALTH TIP

Health is more than the absence of disease. Being healthy is not simply the opposite of being sick. Optimal health means being as healthy as *you* can be. This will be different for each person, and it involves our faith, work, and relationships, along with what what we eat or how much exercise we get. Moving toward better health is a whole-life journey.

— DAILY HEALTH JOURNAL —

Number of steps....................................   O Add 3 servings of vegetables

O Add 2,000 steps   O Add 3 glasses of water

"Stand on your feet."

ACTS 14:5-10

There they continued proclaiming the good news.

—Acts 14:7

AFTER LEAVING ANTIOCH IN PISIDIA, Paul and Barnabas went into the region of Iconium. Despite their experience with the Jewish leaders in Pisidia, they persisted in their strategy of going first to the Jews. Once again many believed, and once again Jewish leaders stirred up trouble. Paul and Barnabas persisted in their mission, but when they were threatened with stoning, they moved on to the cities of Lystra and Derbe, where they "continued proclaiming the good news."

In Lystra they encountered a man born with a physical disability that meant he had never been able to walk. This man listened intently to Paul. Perhaps Paul saw something in the man's expression, or perhaps Paul had a spiritual glimpse into the man's heart. In that moment, Paul saw that faith and health were coming together. When he told the man to stand on his feet, the man did!

Proclaiming good news is healing work, and healing is as much God's call for modern-day disciples as it as in the first century. Not every person is gifted for great oratory or profound teaching, but we also proclaim the good news when we recognize and affirm the gift of faith in each other and are companions to each other in moving toward levels of health and wellness we might never have imagined possible. Who can you walk alongside today?

HEALTH TIP

Small bits of time can contribute to achieving your goals of becoming healthier and stronger. For instance, if you are standing in line in the store, the post office, or anywhere else, use the time to exercise your ankles and calves by doing calf raises. Rise onto your toes and let yourself back down. Gradually lengthen the amount of time you can balance on your toes.

— DAILY HEALTH JOURNAL —

Number of steps................

O Add 2,000 steps

O Add 3 servings of vegetables

O Add 3 glasses of water

Good Intentions Gone Wrong
ACTS 14:11–18

*"We bring you good news, that you should turn
from these worthless things to the living God."*
—Acts 14:15

WHEN PAUL HEALED THE MAN in Lystra who was lame, the crowds who witnessed the healing responding by rapidly forming what we might call a "fan base." They were shouting that Paul and Barnabas were Greek gods in human form—Zeus and Hermes. Even the priests who led worship of these gods believed this erroneous message and came prepared to offer sacrifices to Paul and Barnabas.

Paul and Barnabas wanted nothing of this! They had come to preach the good news of Jesus Christ, not to bring glory to themselves. They wanted no fans; they wanted only to point people toward faith in the true living God who made all of creation. Everything the people in Lystra possessed or experienced came from God, and it was God who deserved praise and thanks. Yet the crowd continued to rally, and Paul and Barnabas had to work hard to keep people from worshiping them rather than God.

"Turn away from worthless things," was the heart of their message. "Turn to God." Our faith, not only for eternal salvation but also for healing and grace in the moments of our days, is in God. Being drawn to the latest rage or a popular gimmick can pull our eyes off of God, from whom everything we have comes. Our health journeys can point us to being true followers of God, rather than people who go along with the crowd.

HEALTH TIP
Stress happens to all of us. Because it can contribute to disease, it's important to be mindful of how to manage stress. Some quick ideas include: make time for your hobbies; keep regular sleeping hours; take mini-breaks—a few minutes, or part of a day; accept that it is okay to say "no" when you need to; keep favorite music handy; keep a gratitude list and add to it every day.

— DAILY HEALTH JOURNAL —

Number of steps............................   ○ Add 3 servings of vegetables
○ Add 2,000 steps   ○ Add 3 glasses of water

Left for Dead

ACTS 14:19-20

But when the disciples surrounded him,
he got up and went into the city.
—Acts 14:20

WE MIGHT THINK THAT PAUL and Barnabas were physically safe in Lystra—even though the people there misunderstood the message cradled by the miracle of healing the man who was lame. But the Jewish leaders who had incited mobs in Antioch and Iconium now arrived in Lystra, and the tide turned quickly. The crowd that was so eager to worship Paul and Barnabas was soon enough convinced to stone them. Paul was stoned, dragged outside the city limits, and left for dead.

But others in Lystra who believed in Jesus did not abandon him. Instead they surrounded Paul, and Luke tells us that Paul got up and went back into the city! Luke does not say that the others carried Paul but that he got up from a stoning brutal enough that he was supposed dead. He went into the city, and he was well enough that the very next day he was able to travel with Barnabas to Derbe.

What a beautiful picture of the healing power of community! When we gather around each other, we give each other a place of belonging, healing touches, a hedge against the discouragements that threaten, and safe passage to the next season of what God calls us to do. Even in our most extreme experiences, when we might be tempted to admit defeat, the people around us can be the ones to help us to our feet and give us a fresh vision of the path to healing and wholeness.

HEALTH TIP

If you're training for a long race—whatever *long* is for you—physical conditioning matters. But long distance runners will say that endurance is at least as emotional as it is physical. When you think about the healthy changes you are working on making, make sure you are staying in good condition emotionally for success. Take a few minutes to concentrate on breathing and reminding yourself of why you have chosen your healthy goals.

--- **DAILY HEALTH JOURNAL** ---

Number of steps ....   O Add 3 servings of vegetables
O Add 2,000 steps   O Add 3 glasses of water

Strength for the Soul
ACTS 14:21-23

*There they strengthened the souls of the
disciples and encouraged them to continue in the faith.*
—Acts 14:22

I N DERBE PAUL AND BARNABAS continued to preach the good news of Jesus. Luke tells us not only that they preached but also that they "made many disciples" (Acts 14:21). They were not preaching in order to be able to say they were doing God's work but to see God at work in changing lives.

At this point, they could have continued in the loop their route had formed and returned to their base in Antioch in Syria. Instead, they retraced their steps to the cities where they had faced so much difficulty. Rather than seeing the hardships as a reason to quit, they thought of them as a way to participate in the kingdom of God. On these return visits, they took steps to be sure the fledgling faith communities in Lystra, Iconium, and Antioch in Pisidia would endure, both by speaking words of encouragement and by appointing leaders in each congregation. Paul and Barnabas didn't look for short-cuts. They kept the long-term view in mind and made the investment necessary for growth and success.

Our own health journeys benefit from these same principles. We live in the good news of God's kingdom even when times are difficult. There is a difference between the quick choice and the right choice, and the changes we seek in well-being come from keeping the long view in mind. Let us strengthen and encourage each other, just as Paul did for the first churches.

HEALTH TIP

Take a few minutes right now and check in with your emotional state. Are you just beginning the day? In the middle of it? Closing it out? Jot down how you feel about the challenges of this day. Then brainstorm two or three small healthy choices you can make for yourself today to be sure that your emotional state remains in balance with the rest of your wellness goals.

— DAILY HEALTH JOURNAL —

Number of steps............................   O Add 3 servings of vegetables

O Add 2,000 steps   O Add 3 glasses of water

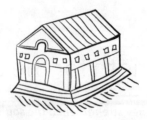

Week Two in Review

IN THIS WEEK'S PICTURES from Paul's first missionary journey, we see boldness and determination. We see healing and grace in hard times. We see communities rising up and gathering around a common purpose of abundant living.

Being on a six-week journey toward wellness puts us in a good position to appreciate lessons from Paul's journeys. How do the traits of boldness and determination manifest in your journey? What healing and grace have you experienced in body and spirit because of the choices and changes you are making in your health habits? What communities are you part of that encourage and strengthen you? In what ways do you see the hope that the kingdom of God brings? In what ways can you journey alongside others also pursuing greater wellness?

Transfer your daily steps in the space below. If you set a goal for all three categories, put checkmarks in the boxes where you reached your goal for each day.

Number of steps	Add 2,000 steps	Add 3 vegetables	Add 3 glasses of water
Day 1	O	O	O
Day 2	O	O	O
Day 3	O	O	O
Day 4	O	O	O
Day 5	O	O	O
Day 6	O	O	O
Day 7	O	O	O

Back to Home Base

ACTS 14:24-28

*From there they sailed back to Antioch, where they had been
commended to the grace of God for the work that they had completed.*
—**Acts 14:26**

AFTER PREACHING ONE LAST time in Perga, Paul and Barnabas went to Attalia, the best harbor in the region, and arranged passage back to Antioch in Syria. The church there, which had sent them out (Acts 13:3), was the first Gentile congregation. The church gathered, no doubt eager to hear news of what Paul and Barnabas had experienced in a region where there were some Jewish synagogues but also many more people who were not Jewish and had no understanding that God had promised a Messiah who would bring them into God's kingdom.

Paul and Barnabas completed the work God had given them to do—for this phase. The book of Acts is only half over at this point, and we know from the chapters that come that both Paul and Barnabas continued with additional missionary journeys, preaching the good news, healing the sick, building relationships, and establishing churches.

Sometimes in our work, and in our pursuit of health, we look too far out at the risk of losing focus on what God asks us to do right now. Paul completed the work. He shared what God had done in opening "a door of faith" (Acts 14:28). Only then did Paul turn his eyes to what came next.

What is God asking you to do right now? Complete the work. Share the door of faith God opened through the experience. Then turn your heart to the next call from God.

HEALTH TIP

While you're concentrating on adding steps, vegetables, and water to your day, also keep in mind that holistic spirituality in your daily life can improve health. Take some time each day to experience your own understanding of spirituality. Try some creative ways to meditate and pray. Identify the moments when you feel the most inner harmony and balance and reflect on what helped bring this about.

— **DAILY HEALTH JOURNAL** —

Number of steps............................   O Add 3 servings of vegetables

O Add 2,000 steps   O Add 3 glasses of water

DAY 16

Paul's Second Journey Begins

ACTS 16:1-5

*He was well spoken of by the
believers in Lystra and Iconium.*

—Acts 16:2

B Y THE BEGINNING OF CHAPTER 16, Paul and Barnabas had agreed to travel separately, and Paul traveled again to Derbe and Lystra, despite the significant opposition there on his previous journey. In Lystra, another important character enters the story—Timothy. Luke tells us that Timothy, a young man at this time, was "well spoken of." In letters that Paul wrote to Timothy years later, we learn that his mother, Eunice, and grandmother, Lois, were Jewish women who believed in Jesus. Eunice taught Timothy the Scriptures beginning when he was a small child (2 Timothy 1:5, 3:15).

Paul saw something in Timothy that prompted him to take the young man under his wing as Barnabas had done for him. He prepared him for a role as a leader. Timothy went on to travel and minister alongside Paul, and years later, when Timothy was more experienced and mature, Paul left him in charge of the growing church in Ephesus.

Our ministries are not our own. The meaning we find in our callings is not for us alone. The well-being we shape and guard is not for us alone. We all bring gifts to our interactions, and together we live in and share the good news of God's healing work in our lives. Paul's example with Timothy and others challenges us to discern the potential in others and help to bring them into the wholeness God wants for all of us.

HEALTH TIP

Healthy self-esteem is essential to a holistic sense of health in all the dimensions of life. Who are the children in your life? Children listen and watch for cues to see what others think about them and may internalize these feelings. Help children develop healthy attitudes about themselves and the world around them. Avoid comparing one child to another. Give children tasks that are neither too easy nor too difficult, and offer honest praise and encouragement.

— DAILY HEALTH JOURNAL —

Number of steps............................   O Add 3 servings of vegetables

O Add 2,000 steps   O Add 3 glasses of water

A Plea for Help
ACTS 16:6-10

*During the night Paul had a vision: there stood a man of Macedonia
pleading with him and saying, "Come over to Macedonia and help us."*
—Acts 16:9

WITH SILAS AND TIMOTHY, Paul traveled through the region of Galatia preaching. In today's verses, we see that they were constantly discerning where God wanted them to go next. The Holy Spirit kept them out of the area known as Asia at the time. Next they considered the region of Bithynia, but the Spirit of Jesus said no. The remaining option, from a geographic perspective, was to go Troas, and this is what they did. However, Troas was a seaport, so they could go no farther without more specific purpose.

At last God made the plan clear by sending Paul a vision of a man pleading for them to help in Macedonia. Immediately they made plans to cross the Mediterranean Sea into the Macedonia region of Greece. (In verse 10, Luke begins to use the word *we* rather than *they*, indicating that he had joined Paul's band of traveling missionaries.)

Perhaps you can identify with the group's eagerness both to serve as God calls you and to find direction on your journey toward greater wellness. Notice that the obvious choice was not always God's calling. Because Paul did not press ahead with his own plans, but sought God's guidance, he was in the right place to respond promptly to the plea for help in Macedonia. When we want to hurl ahead with our own plans, this story reminds us that the right choices may take time to discern but also put us in the right place to serve others.

HEALTH TIP

Substance abuse issues are becoming a public health crisis, and the roots begin early. If you have children in your life, talk to them about addiction. Become knowledgeable yourself and then talk with your children about how alcohol and drugs can be harmful. Don't give long lectures. Listen to questions and answer them—or promise to find out the answers. Most of all, examine your own habits with alcohol and drugs. Actions speak louder than words.

— DAILY HEALTH JOURNAL —

Number of steps ....   ○ Add 3 servings of vegetables
○ Add 2,000 steps   ○ Add 3 glasses of water

On to Macedonia

ACTS 16:11-15

The Lord opened her heart to listen eagerly to what was said by Paul.
—Acts 16:14

PHILIPPI WAS A ROMAN COLONY, military outpost, and commercial center. The city had a very small Jewish population. In fact, it did not have even the ten married men required to form a synagogue. Without this house of worship, a "place of prayer" was established along the river. On the first Sabbath in Philippi, Paul sought out the gathering, where he found not only people who shared his Jewish heritage but also Gentiles drawn to God.

Lydia, who ran a thriving operation of selling expensive purple cloth, was one of the people at the river. Luke tells us that the Lord opened her heart. Lydia believed, and her entire household—which would have included her servants—were baptized into their new faith.

"Stay in my home," Lydia said to Paul. Thus began a relationship where Lydia extended hospitality not only to Paul at the time of their meeting but to the church that resulted from his evangelism (Acts 16:40).

We might think God is more likely to change our lives in a dramatic event. This certainly happened to Paul in Acts 9. In Lydia's story, however, we see the importance of responding to God's nudging with eagerness even when it comes in less dramatic circumstances. This is true even in the changes that come to our health through small choices and gradual shifts in our habits. Even in the small things God opens our hearts to new life.

HEALTH TIP

One way to experience holistic spirituality and to find meaning where you least expect it is to leave room in your daily life for events or encounters to unfold naturally. Lingering a few minutes longer in conversation or allowing some breathing room between activities can allow you to make connections or form plans that will support your overall life goals for better wellness.

— DAILY HEALTH JOURNAL —

Number of steps ....

○ Add 2,000 steps

○ Add 3 servings of vegetables

○ Add 3 glasses of water

Money and Health

ACTS 16:16-23

But Paul, very much annoyed, turned and said to the spirit,
"I order you in the name of Jesus Christ to come out of her."
And it came out that very hour.

—Acts 16:18

A **GIRL BEGAN TO FOLLOW PAUL,** crying out that he spoke for the Most High God. What she said was not untrue, but that anyone should regard her as a source of truth began to perturb Paul. She was a fortune-teller slave who earned a good living for her owners by what she predicted based on an evil spirit. Mingling her proclamations with Paul's preaching was sure to cause confusion about the message of salvation. So one day Paul had enough, and he turned around and ordered the spirit out of the young woman.

Her healing was immediate—and infuriating to her owners, who now would make no money from her supposed ability. The owners were more concerned with their loss of income than either truth or the well-being of another human being. They successfully agitated the crowds by pointing out that visitors to Philippi were Jews coming in with their strange anti-Roman customs. Paul and Silas ended up beaten and jailed because of their act of putting into action a gospel of healing.

Healing costs something. Even pursuing our own healing means giving up habits or relationships that harm us over the long term. How much more difficult it can be to pay the cost of bringing wholeness to others when the cost affects our own finances or well-being. But do we want to be like the slave owners who thought only of their own interests, or like Paul and Silas who demonstrated God's values?

HEALTH TIP

Does it sometimes seem like clutter takes over your life—your cabinets, desk, calendar, and even the room where you relax? Many people find wellness in physically decluttering so that what they have around them are the things that really matter. We can also work on decluttering our minds to make room for what matters—including the possibility of an encounter with God that leads to a deeper understanding of what it means to be healthy.

--- DAILY HEALTH JOURNAL ---

Number of steps............................ ○ Add 3 servings of vegetables
○ Add 2,000 steps ○ Add 3 glasses of water

A Night in Jail

ACTS 16:24-34

*About midnight Paul and Silas were singing hymns to God,
and the prisoners were listening to them.*

—Acts 16:25

AFTER A FLOGGING, PAUL and Silas were fastened in chains to the most secure part of the Roman prison. Imagine the physical toll this took, and the deep darkness of the night. On the outside, perhaps Luke and Timothy were keeping watch until morning, when they might attempt to have their friends released, or at least see them. But in the prison, Paul and Silas were praying and singing.

In a moment when they had every reason to despair, they did not. In a moment when they had every reason to surrender to exhaustion of body and spirit, they did not. They prayed and sang—and not just under their breath. They were loud enough that other prisoners were listening. The story that follows is one of the most famous in the book of Acts. An earthquake shook the foundations of the building, doors flew open, chains came loose. Now the jailer was despairing to the brink of suicide, because he would be held responsible for the prisoners who would undoubtedly escape. Paul called out, "Do not harm yourself, for we are all here" (Acts 16:28). The man believed the gospel message that night, and his entire household was baptized.

What a contrast between the inner resources of Paul and Silas and how quickly the jailer gave himself over to his fate. In times of well-being it is important to nurture the inner sense of meaning and purpose that will sustain us even in the most difficult times.

HEALTH TIP

Discouragement is a health issue. Lingering illness, a financial setback, a fractured relationship, a challenging child—these things and more cause discouragement which can easily progress to anxiety and full-blow stress. Is it possible to find hope even in discouragement? Building healthy habits and relationships when times are good strengthens our resiliency for when times are more challenging. With resiliency, it's possible to see past the dark time to renewed life on the other side.

— **DAILY HEALTH JOURNAL** —

Number of steps .... ⃝ Add 3 servings of vegetables
⃝ Add 2,000 steps ⃝ Add 3 glasses of water

Terms of Release

ACTS 16:35-40

After leaving the prison they went to Lydia's home; and when they had seen and encouraged the brothers and sisters there, they departed.
—**Acts 16:40**

O FFICIALLY, PAUL AND SILAS were released in the morning. Unashamed of the circumstances that had gotten them jailed, and calling on the Roman citizenship that should have precluded their mistreatment, Paul insisted that the magistrates so eager to do away with them should come and release them personally. Clearing his name would make the environment safer for the Christian believers of Philippi, who would no longer be associated with a publicly arrested criminal or presumed to also be criminals.

The magistrates did as Paul asked, but with their apology came a request that Paul leave the city. Paul did leave, but not as immediately as the magistrates might have liked. Instead, Paul and Silas went to Lydia's house, where members of the newborn church were gathered. Once again we see Paul's concern not for his own welfare—leaving directly would have been the surest way not to fall out of favor with the crowds and city officials again—but his thought for how to encourage his brothers and sisters in the gospel. Only after he had done this did he leave Philippi.

People matter. Even if his visit was brief, Paul took the detour to reassure new believers of his well-being and their safety. How easy it is to focus on our own circumstances, or our experiences of being treated unfairly, without also lifting our eyes to the effect on other people. Who might you reassure today?

HEALTH TIP

A daily dose of laughter may eliminate some of the stress that contributes to heart disease and other medical conditions. Did you know that 20 seconds of laughter raises your heart rate for the next few minutes? People who show a strong sense of humor tend to be less anxious than people who laugh less. Let your silly inner child come out to play. Boost your immune system by having an old-fashioned belly laugh!

— DAILY HEALTH JOURNAL —

Number of steps......................   O Add 3 servings of vegetables
O Add 2,000 steps   O Add 3 glasses of water

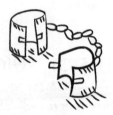

Week Three in Review

AS THIS WEEK OPENED, WE FOUND PAUL completing his first missionary journey. One phase of his ministry had come to an end, and he faced new challenges in new places with new companions. We saw him being intentional about seeking God's guidance and undertaking work that would not bring glory to himself but that would sink roots of faith into new people and new cities with a healing message of wholeness.

You've reached the half-way point in *Walking with Paul*. What new roots have you found yourself sinking? In what ways have you been challenged to notice the people around you and what effect you might have on them? In what ways have you discerned God's guidance and call on your journey to unite your faith and your health? Take a few minutes to jot down some of the ideas that come to your mind. Spend a few minutes in prayer being grateful for God's presence on your journey. If appropriate, adjust your health habit goals as you embark on the second half of the program.

Transfer your daily steps in the space below. If you set a goal for all three categories, put checkmarks in the boxes where you reached your goal for each day.

Number of steps	Add 2,000 steps	Add 3 vegetables	Add 3 glasses of water
Day 1	O	O	O
Day 2	O	O	O
Day 3	O	O	O
Day 4	O	O	O
Day 5	O	O	O
Day 6	O	O	O
Day 7	O	O	O

"This is the Messiah."

ACTS 17:1-4

And Paul went in, as was his custom, and on three
sabbath days argued with them from the scriptures.
—Acts 17:2

AFTER LEAVING PHILIPPI, Paul traveled a road that crossed present-day northern Greece from east to west, going through several cities spaced about a day's walk apart—around 30 miles. This brought him to Thessalonica, the largest city in Macedonia and about 100 miles from Philippi. We have already seen that Paul's custom was to preach first to his Jewish brothers and sisters who shared his hope of the Messiah whom God would send for the salvation of the world.

Paul's approach was not to introduce some new-fangled notion the Jews had never heard of, but rather to begin with their own belief in the coming Messiah and the evidence in the holy writings they held dear. For instance, this may have included discussing Psalm 22, Isaiah 53, and Zechariah 12 to illustrate that the Messiah the prophets wrote about would indeed suffer and die.

The result was that some Jews believed in Jesus the Messiah, and along with them Greeks who had been listening to the reasoned arguments. Luke makes special note that "leading women" also believed and could influence others.

Paul followed his usual habit. He knew the task of preaching Jesus the Messiah would not be accomplished overnight. It required a sustained, systematic approach that moved him steadily toward his goal. Our health benefits from a similar approach—information rooted in trustworthy evidence and a sustained patience that moves us toward our goals.

HEALTH TIP

We all know that nutritious foods are better for our health and energy. Yet planning what to eat seems to be a hard habit to form. If you normally eat lunch away from home, you can take control by planning ahead for leftovers from last night's dinner. It's likely to be healthier than eating out of a vending machine or grabbing fast food. Developing a habit of planning ahead removes temptations that undermine your goals.

— DAILY HEALTH JOURNAL —

Number of steps............................   O Add 3 servings of vegetables

O Add 2,000 steps   O Add 3 glasses of water

DAY 23

Ruffians in the Marketplace

ACTS 17:5-9

But as the Jews became jealous, and with the help of some ruffians in the marketplaces they formed a mob and set the city in an uproar.
—Acts 17:5

FOR A MOMENT, LOOK AT EVENTS in Thessalonica from the viewpoint of the Jewish synagogue leaders. A stranger came, preached, and began drawing a following—from the very people the Jewish leaders thought should be listening to *their* message. Jealousy is an intense emotion, entangled with distrust and possessiveness. Jealousy often prompts us to express ourselves in ways that hurt others. In this case, jealous Jewish leaders formed an alliance with ruffians in the marketplace based on the lowest common denominator: distrust for these outsiders.

A mob formed, and when they couldn't find Paul and Silas, they grabbed whoever they could and dragged them before the city officials. There they trotted out the argument that Jesus somehow threatened the emperor. "There is another king named Jesus" (Acts 17: 7). The city officials would not dare ignore such an accusation, because if it proved true, their own futures would be on the chopping block.

Have you ever been jealous enough that you made ridiculous statements? Or accused someone of ridiculous behavior? Our health pilgrimages are not exempt from the power of jealousy. If someone else is losing weight faster, are you jealous? If someone else seems to have more success at work or in relationships, are you jealous? Recognize that jealousy may be a sign that you should turn your thoughts inward to understand yourself better before you take your feelings out on someone else in the wrong ways.

HEALTH TIP

Depression is persistent feelings of sadness, isolation, discouragement, or hopelessness. It affects all the dimensions of a person's life. Symptoms include feelings of worthlessness, difficulty sleeping or eating, decreased energy, and difficulty concentrating. If you experience symptoms for longer than two weeks, or the symptoms make it hard for you to function in your daily life, your primary care provider is a good place to start to get help.

— DAILY HEALTH JOURNAL —

Number of steps ....   O Add 3 servings of vegetables

O Add 2,000 steps   O Add 3 glasses of water

Disturbing the Balance
ACTS 17:10-15

These Jews were more receptive than those in Thessalonica,
for they welcomed the message very eagerly and examined the
scriptures every day to see whether these things were so.
—Acts 17:11

PAUL RECOGNIZED THE TIME had come to leave Thessalonica, perhaps at the behest of the synagogue. We have not seen him walk away from his calling or custom simply becomes circumstances become difficult. In Beroea, Luke tells us, "These Jews were more receptive than those in Thessalonica." The Beroeans are famous in the biblical record for examining Paul's claims in light of the Scriptures—the same approach Paul himself had used in Thessalonica.

But trouble followed Paul even when things were going well. The Thessalonicans weren't satisfied to have Paul out of their city; they wanted him out of Beroea as well. So once again the believers sent Paul on to safety.

The gospel of Jesus was good news, and Paul demonstrated the ways it was consistent with the Jewish Scriptures. So why was it so hard for the Jewish leaders to accept good news? That's a question worth asking about ourselves as well. How often is our first impulse to respond on the basis of what we already have decided is true, rather than what we could learn by listening and examining questions more deeply?

Sometimes what we need for better health is to upset the apple cart and open our minds and spirits to understanding truths to which we have closed ourselves off—truths about ourselves, and truth about where real health comes from.

HEALTH TIP

Did you know 200 different viruses can give you a cold? When someone sneezes, germs fly out at a ferocious speed looking for someone to land on. Preventively, be sure to wash your hands often, keep hands away from your face, and get adequate rest. If you are the person with a cold, cough or sneeze into a tissue or the elbow of your arm to help reduce spread of germs.

— DAILY HEALTH JOURNAL —

Number of steps.........................   O Add 3 servings of vegetables

O Add 2,000 steps   O Add 3 glasses of water

Tentmaking
ACTS 18:1-3

Because he was of the same trade, he stayed with them,
and they worked together—by trade they were tentmakers.
—Acts 18:3

PAUL TRAVELED ON TO ATHENS and then to Corinth. Up until now, the book of Acts has said nothing of Paul's finances. In Corinth, we discover he was a tentmaker. He was a well-educated Jew who had studied with a famous rabbi, but even rabbinical students needed a trade, and apparently Paul learned to make tents. It may be that he arrived in Corinth short of funds after a long journey and this is why Luke mentions his trade. Aquila and Priscilla previously lived in Rome, until the Emperor Claudius decreed that all the Jews must leave the city because they seemed to be at the heart of riots about Christ. Imagine the conversations Paul, Aquila and Priscilla might have had about being chased out of town because they stirred up riots!

It seems that Paul sought out his new friends. Luke tells us that Paul "went to see them." They welcomed him—"he stayed with them"—and perhaps part of their welcome was offering to take him into their work so his needs would be provided for. Perhaps someone had recommended Paul to Aquila and Priscilla, a demonstration of community in action and the kinds of connections that can bring benefit and create lifelong friendships. This picture of Paul gives us a glimpse into the value he placed on community with others who shared common work and goals and challenges us to consider how we, too, can build a community of wellness.

HEALTH TIP

Protecting your sleep is essential to well-being. We may go through seasons where uninterrupted sleep is difficult, such as parenting young children or extended caregiving. Even at these times, a simple stretching routine before bedtime can help you fall asleep more easily and sleep more comfortably. Look for a brief routine that targets neck, shoulders, back, hips, and legs in gentle stretches. Pair the stretching with deep breathing for even more benefit.

— DAILY HEALTH JOURNAL —

Number of steps ....   ○ Add 3 servings of vegetables
○ Add 2,000 steps   ○ Add 3 glasses of water

Meeting the Neighbors

ACTS 18:7-8

Then he left the synagogue and went to the house
of a man named Titius Justus, a worshiper of God.
—Acts 18:7

PAUL CONTINUED HIS USUAL CUSTOM of speaking to Jews in the synagogue (Acts 18:4). One day he left the synagogue and went next door to a man who was not a Jew but who worshiped God. The people with whom Paul had most in common—Jews—"opposed and reviled him" (Acts 18:6), and those with whom he had the least in common—Romans—received him with welcome.

If we're honest, many of us do not know our neighbors, at least not well enough to feel at ease in their homes. Yet, as for Paul, people who are not like us may be our nearest neighbors. One of the important dimensions in whole-life health is the relationships we have with friends and family. If we cut ourselves off from people who may become our friends because we assume we will have nothing in common with them, we lose out both on the enrichment we might receive from the relationship and, even ore important, on the opportunity to offer the gift of friendship to someone who may need it.

Notice the people around you today, whether in your place of work, on your errands, or the neighbors who literally live on either side of you. How well do you know the people around you? What simple gesture might you offer that opens the door to conversation and friendship that might draw you together as co-journeyers on the road to a deeper understanding of what it means to be whole and well?

HEALTH TIP

Why exercise? Here are some quick benefits of exercise: it improves the cardio-respiratory system, builds and maintains muscle strength, helps manage weight, prevents or manages high blood pressure, aids in good sleep, and relieves tension. Exercise doesn't mean everyone must become a marathoner or body-builder. It simply means moving more and getting your heart rate up for a few minutes every day. Finding ways that *you* enjoy moving is the important thing.

— DAILY HEALTH JOURNAL —

Number of steps ....   O Add 3 servings of vegetables

O Add 2,000 steps   O Add 3 glasses of water

DAY 27

"Do not be afraid."

ACTS 18:9-11

One night the Lord said to Paul in a vision,
"Do not be afraid, but speak and do not be silent."
—Acts 18:9

PAUL ONCE AGAIN HAD success in his ministry and once again found himself at odds with Jewish leaders. Luke tells us they "reviled" him, a strong word for strong emotion. We can well imagine that the tension worsened when Crispus, the official of the synagogue, became a Christian (Acts 18:8).

If you were Paul, wouldn't you be thinking about the ugliness that resulted when Jewish leaders decided you were too much of a threat to tolerate? He'd been chased out of one city after another and even once had been been left for dead after a stoning. His calling was clear and his commitment unquestioned. Still, it's easy to imagine moments of discouragement. Maybe it was time to leave Corinth before things got worse.

Perhaps it was in one of these times, with Paul lying awake on his bed, that the Lord came to him in a vision of reassurance. "Do not be afraid, but speak and do not be silent; for I am with you, and no one will lay a hand on you to harm you" (Acts 18:9-10).

What an encouragement that God does not abandon us in our discouragement. Paul rose up and found the endurance to remain in Corinth for a year and a half, holding steadfast to God's calling for him. This same God remains with you in times of discouragement with assurance that you matter to God.

HEALTH TIP

When you sleep for a stretch of hours, your body fasts. When you wake, you need to break the fast ("breakfast") in a way that fuels your body and brain. A healthy breakfast improves memory and creativity and can reduce stress. Include carbohydrates for energy and protein to keep you feeling satisfied until your next meal. A good breakfast starts your day in a healthy way and immediately moves you toward your daily goal.

— DAILY HEALTH JOURNAL —

Number of steps ....

O Add 2,000 steps

O Add 3 servings of vegetables

O Add 3 glasses of water

Visiting Ephesus

ACTS 18:18-21

But on taking leave of them, he said,
"I will return to you, if God wills."
—Acts 18:21

WHEN **PAUL LEFT CORINTH** after a year and a half, he took with him Priscilla and Aquila and sailed for Syria. At Ephesus, another city where Paul spent considerable time during the years of his ministry, of course he went first to the synagogue. We would expect nothing less! In fact, this time the Jews asked if Paul might stay longer, but he declined—with the hope that he would return someday.

When he sailed, however, he left Priscilla and Aquila in Ephesus to lead the ministry. After spending a year and a half living and working and ministering together, Paul was confident in their ability. Priscilla and Aquila went on to prove both their gentle ways and their authority when Apollos came to town and spoke boldly in the synagogue—but not quite accurately (Acts 18:26). They took him aside for private instruction, and he matured into a persuasive leader.

Paul was able to let go. He maintained a warm relationship with the church in Ephesus, both returning when the time was right and writing the letter that we know as the book of Ephesians. But for this season, he let go and left his tentmaking friends to lead the ministry.

Sometimes we, too, need to let go and affirm the gifts of others. Perhaps this is the right time for you to consider this question. Is your season of ministry shifting? For our own wellness, at times we must step back or explore new opportunities and entrust our ministries to God.

HEALTH TIP

If you are caring for someone else, remember to care for yourself as well. No matter how strong and loving you are, you need rest, nutrition, and movement as regular parts of your day. Other healing influences may be all around you—art, nature, music, literature, spiritual habits. Even in brief moments and small ways, welcome healing into your own life as you offer it to someone else.

— DAILY HEALTH JOURNAL —

Number of steps ....   ○ Add 3 servings of vegetables
○ Add 2,000 steps   ○ Add 3 glasses of water

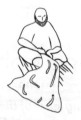

Week Four in Review

DURING WEEK FOUR, we have seen Paul's ministry expand and deepen. We've seen friendship, co-laboring, discouragement, and reassurance. And through it all we have seen steadfastness when distraction might have been the easier road.

What parallels can you see between the ways Paul's ministry developed as he visited Philippi, Thessalonica, Beroea, Corinth, and Ephesus and how your understanding of your journey toward wellness has developed? Perhaps you have found encouragement for times of discouragement. Perhaps you have looked around and seen the people who share your goals or to whom you can offer friendship. Perhaps you have sensed an expanding and deepening call to a form of ministry for yourself.

This is a good time to reflect on these questions and jot down insights. You might want to choose a friend—someone also on the journey to greater wellness—to share your thoughts with and welcome a perspective other than your own as you seek clarity for decisions you face.

Transfer your daily steps in the space below. If you set a goal for all three categories, put checkmarks in the boxes where you reached your goal for each day.

Number of steps	Add 2,000 steps	Add 3 vegetables	Add 3 glasses of water
Day 1	O	O	O
Day 2	O	O	O
Day 3	O	O	O
Day 4	O	O	O
Day 5	O	O	O
Day 6	O	O	O
Day 7	O	O	O

Back to the Base

ACTS 18:22-23

There he departed and went from place to place through the region of Galatia and Phrygia, strengthening the disciples.
—**Acts 18:23**

AS PAUL WOUND DOWN his second major journey as a missionary, he chose to visit Jerusalem. The city where Jesus had died and been raised to life again was still the center of Christianity. Although Paul's encounter with Jesus Christ on the road to Damascus, in Acts 9, happened apart from the disciples who had known and followed Jesus in and around Jerusalem, he recognized the importance of maintaining a positive relationship with Christian leaders in Jerusalem.

Then Paul continued on to Antioch and the church that had first laid hands on him to send him out as a missionary. After that visit, which no doubt included many reports from the years he was away, Paul left on what we know as his third major missionary journey. This included going back to the places he had visited while traveling with Silas for the purpose of "strengthening the disciples."

Paul was in a time of transition between his second journey and his third, and he seemed quite thoughtful about his decision to tend to important relationships. He reminds us of the value of being intentional during times of transition, whether the changes are related to work, family, household location, or shifts in calling. It's easy to feel like we bounce from one thing to another without being in control. Even a few moments and a few deep breaths can help restore our priorities and enable us to be intentional about what comes next.

HEALTH TIP

What pieces of your life influence what you should discuss with your doctor? All of it! Stress at work may contribute to disease. Your emotions may influence how well you cope. Pain in your feet might make exercise difficult. You might think that many things are not worth mentioning to a health care provider, but doctors cannot help with what they don't know. Aim for an open, honest relationship with your doctor.

— **DAILY HEALTH JOURNAL** —

Number of steps............................   O Add 3 servings of vegetables

O Add 2,000 steps   O Add 3 glasses of water

Paul's Third Journey Begins

ACTS 19:8-10

*He entered the synagogue and for three months spoke out boldly,
and argued persuasively about the kingdom of God.*
—Acts 19:8

AT LAST PAUL HAS THE extended time in Ephesus that he seemed to want. For three months, Luke tells us, Paul spoke boldly in the synagogue about the kingdom of God. At the outset of his ministry, Jesus announced that "the kingdom of God has come near" (Mark 1:14), and used parables to teach what the kingdom of God was like. In recognizing Jesus as the Messiah, Paul embraced the truth that the kingdom had come.

Some resisted Paul's teaching, of course. At this point, Paul switched gears. Rather than continue to argue with the resisters, he took those who were receptive to another location where he could teach them. For an additional two years, he continued teaching about the kingdom of God.

Yet the message did not remain only in Ephesus. Luke wrote, "All the residents of Asia, both Jews and Greeks, heard the word of the Lord" (Acts 19:10). Out of this time of ministry in Ephesus, churches were born all across the region. Paul was bold, persistent, and strategic, and over time the results were indisputable.

Our response to God's calling has similar potential. Do we embrace the purpose? Do we consider where we might have the most effect? Do we wait patiently for the Spirit of God to work? Whether you are answering the call to pursue better health or considering a new form of service, remember what Paul teaches us by his example.

HEALTH TIP

The first steps in changing a health habit are the hardest. It can feel overwhelming to look up at the mountain and see how far we have to go. But every journey begins with putting one foot in front of the other. Small steps add up to cover the distance of the journey, just as small changes in our health habits add up to change the direction and take us closer to our goals.

— DAILY HEALTH JOURNAL —

Number of steps ....   ○ Add 3 servings of vegetables

○ Add 2,000 steps   ○ Add 3 glasses of water

No Fake Jesus

ACTS 19:11-20

God did extraordinary miracles through Paul, so that when the handkerchiefs or aprons that had touched his skin were brought to the sick, their diseases left them.

—Acts 19:11–12

PAUL IS KNOWN AS A GREAT ORATOR, teacher, and writer of much of the New Testament, but he also was a vessel for the healing reality of the gospel. Luke tells us that "God did extraordinary miracles through Paul." Something as simple as a handkerchief that touched Paul's skin and then the sick person resulted in healing.

Perhaps Luke takes care to identify God as the source of these miracles because Ephesus was a focal point for magicians, including some Jewish, who were anxious to demonstrate their own power with secret incantations. Paul, of course, had no gimmick. God's power flowed through him. Eventually, though, others latched on to the idea that they could also claim to do miracles in the name of this Jesus as a form of incantation. Their efforts met defeat. They were humiliated, and rather than draw attention to their own powers, they pointed at the power of God.

This led to many people becoming believers in Jesus, and the secret records of incantations and spells piled up ready for a bon fire. This was akin to burning money; the books of magic would have been worth a great deal if the owners had simply kept them secret.

Often we think we need some kind of gimmick in order to do something that matters. But Paul's example shows us that making ourselves available to God, for God's glory and not our own, has the potential to affect the lives of more people than we can count.

HEALTH TIP

This program has challenged you to add 2,000 steps a day to the baseline you began with. Perhaps by now you are ready to take it up another notch. Carrying small weights as you walk adds aerobic value to your exercise. You can use small hand weights and choose the weight you're comfortable with. Or, you can fill a couple of bottles with water and carry those with you on a walk.

— DAILY HEALTH JOURNAL —

Number of steps............................ ○ Add 3 servings of vegetables

○ Add 2,000 steps ○ Add 3 glasses of water

Eyes on Jerusalem

ACTS 19:21-22

Paul resolved in the Spirit to go through
Macedonia and Achaia and then go on to Jerusalem.

—Acts 19:21

T'S EASY TO SKIP OVER short passages like this one, only a verse or two that read like entries in a travelogue. We want to know what exciting events happened where Paul was, and what will happen in the next place he goes. Does reading about how he got from one place to another really matter?

These two simple verses remind us about several things. First Paul made decisions "in the Spirit"—waiting on God's direction. With God's guidance, he decided to go through Macedonia and Achaia, and then to Jerusalem. Second, he thought beyond the immediate moment to what the greater purpose was for his work. He was a Roman citizen who lived in the expansive Roman Empire of the time. He saw the influence and reality of Roman rule everywhere he went. And he knew that even those who ruled Rome were loved by God and would be welcome in God's kingdom. And third, we see him once again making sure his fellow-laborers were dispatched to where their work would have value. Timothy, of course, was the young man Paul took under his wing early in his second journey. Now we learn of Erastus as well, so Paul continued to expand his team of ministers.

These are three practical lessons for us: Seek God's guidance; consider the greater purpose; and invite others into the journey of answering God's call.

HEALTH TIP

Eating disorders are on the rise among teenage girls and young women. They fall into two main categories. Anorexia nervosa manifests in a pursuit to be thin, even if the woman already is very thin, and taking in too few calories for healthy nutrition. Bulimia, in contrast, includes binge eating and them self-induced vomiting or laxatives. Both are eating disorders that require medical attention and careful monitoring.

— DAILY HEALTH JOURNAL —

Number of steps............................   ○ Add 3 servings of vegetables
○ Add 2,000 steps   ○ Add 3 glasses of water

Burning Midnight Oil

ACTS 20:7-12

But Paul went down, and bending over him took him in his arms,
and said, "Do not be alarmed, for his life is in him."

—Acts 20:10

PAUL IS ONCE AGAIN ON THE ROAD with Luke and others, headed for Jerusalem, and stops for a week's visit in the seaport of Troas. On the Sabbath, the believers gathered. Paul was leaving the next day, so time was valuable, and he preached late into the night in an upstairs room. Luke does not tell us what Paul spoke about that night, but he does tell us that a young man named Eutychus, perhaps a young teenager, was sitting in an open window and dozed off some time after midnight. He might have been at the window because the room was crowded and warm from the lamps, making it difficult to remain alert. Eutychus fell three floors to the ground outside. No doubt others thundered down the stairs to reach him as quickly as possible, but they were too late. They picked him up, dead.

Notice how smoothly Paul transitioned from preaching and teaching to demonstrating the gospel through healing. He bent over Eutychus and spoke reassurance—he was alive!

We might think that this dramatic event would have broken up the gathering for the night. But just as smoothly as he transitioned to healing, Paul moved back to speaking.

Paul was always willing to talk about Jesus, and over food, conversation continued until dawn. The way he integrated healing into his teaching reminds us that the healing work of the gospel is not something pushed to the side, but something to hold front and center.

HEALTH TIP

Too many people don't have regular primary care providers, and when they get sick they have nowhere to go. Even if you have a doctor but need to change for some reason, get to know a new provider while you are well. Establish a relationship that lets the doctor understand what is important to you and that allows the doctor to know what "healthy" looks like for you.

— DAILY HEALTH JOURNAL —

Number of steps........................   O Add 3 servings of vegetables

O Add 2,000 steps   O Add 3 glasses of water

Six weeks of devotions for body and spirit **53**

Eager for Jerusalem

ACTS 20:17-24

"But I do not count my life of any value to myself, if only I may finish my course and the ministry that I received from the Lord Jesus."

—Acts 20:24

STILL ON HIS WAY TO JERUSALEM, Paul made another brief stop. His itinerary did not allow him to go to Ephesus, where no doubt he would have been drawn into an extended visit, because he wanted to be in Jerusalem in time for the feast of Pentecost. But because he was reasonably close, in Miletus, Paul asked the elders of the Ephesian church to meet him there. After Jerusalem, Paul intended to go to Rome. The tenderness of his encouragement to the elders from Ephesus suggests he knew he would not see them again, and in fact, he says this outright (Acts 20:25). Paul was saying his goodbyes to people he cared for deeply. It must have been an exquisite occasion for all of them.

Paul said he was "captive to the Spirit" (Acts 20:22). The danger in Jerusalem was unknown but certain; everywhere Paul went, the Holy Spirit told him that imprisonment and persecution awaited him (Acts 17:23), yet he was compelled forward into his own discomfort for the sake of the greater glory for God.

When circumstances become difficult, quitting starts to look attractive. This is true whether the challenge is in our work, relationships, or health habits. "If only I may finish my course," Paul said. When God calls us toward a choice, and we are "captive to the Spirit," we know that we are doing something worthwhile even when it becomes difficult.

HEALTH TIP

What does it mean to you to live in the moment, or in the present? Many people focus on regrets from the past or uncertainties of the future and thus miss the beauty of the moments before them. Take a few minutes to breathe in deeply, saying, "This is the day" and then exhale and say, "that the Lord made." Find the calm that comes from being present in the moment.

— **DAILY HEALTH JOURNAL** —

Number of steps ....   ○ Add 3 servings of vegetables

○ Add 2,000 steps   ○ Add 3 glasses of water

Support the Weak

ACTS 20:32-38

"In all this I have given you an example that by such work we must support the weak, remembering the words of the Lord Jesus, for he himself said, 'It is more blessed to give than to receive.'"

—**Acts 20:35**

PAUL WAS HEADED TOWARD persecution when he headed to Jerusalem this time, but he also knew that the congregation in Ephesus would face difficulties of its own. This would include hostility from those outside the church but also people within the church who would introduce wrong teaching (Acts 20:30). So Paul's parting words to the Ephesian elders include an exhortation to remain alert. And then he gave them to God's care and grace. Life would not be perfect—far from it. But God's care and grace would sustain them (Acts 20:32).

And finally, Paul reminded his friends to remember those in need. Paul had worked as a tentmaker to support himself and the companions who traveled with him. He pointed to his example not to gain accolades but to demonstrate that everyone, including leaders, must cultivate generosity and awareness of those around us who have particular needs that we can help meet. "Support the weak" applies on many levels of our daily lives. It boils down to caring for each other with a generous spirit.

Then the elders prayed for Paul. They wept. They hugged and kissed him. Along with an exhortation to generosity, we see a picture of heartfelt, deep Christian fellowship. Think of the power of that combination—generosity and fellowship. Such expressions of care go a long way.

HEALTH TIP

Diabetes is on the rise in the United States. Complications from the disease are serious and even life-threatening. The type of diabetes most likely to occur in adults is related to lifestyle—nutrition and movement choices—that impairs the body's ability to turn food into fuel for energy. The next time you see your doctor, talk about your blood sugar levels and what changes you should consider to prevent or manage diabetes.

— DAILY HEALTH JOURNAL —

Number of steps.............................   O Add 3 servings of vegetables
O Add 2,000 steps   O Add 3 glasses of water

Six weeks of devotions for body and spirit **55**

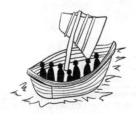

Week Five in Review

IN WEEK FIVE WE HAVE SEEN Paul building and tending relationships, being intentional during transitions, discerning long-term goals, and opening himself to genuine, tender fellowship with other believers.

How would these experiences of Paul's translate into your life? What relationships would you like to tend and deepen? What transitions might you be facing in the weeks or months ahead? What goals or decisions are on your heart for which you could seek to be "captive to the Spirit" as Paul was?

All of these questions bear on your overall well-being. They help us manage stress and contribute to finding meaning and purpose in our lives, which in turn has the potential to improve some chronic physical conditions. Bringing body and spirit together in purpose and service is a health habit!

Transfer your daily steps in the space below. If you set a goal for all three categories, put checkmarks in the boxes where you reached your goal for each day.

Number of steps	Add 2,000 steps	Add 3 vegetables	Add 3 glasses of water
Day 1	O	O	O
Day 2	O	O	O
Day 3	O	O	O
Day 4	O	O	O
Day 5	O	O	O
Day 6	O	O	O
Day 7	O	O	O

Another Farewell

ACTS 21:1-15

We looked up the disciples and stayed there for seven days.
—Acts 21:4

PAUL'S DAYS DURING THIS SEASON were full of goodbyes. In the space of a few verses we read that he spent a week in Tyre, a day in Ptolemais, and several days in Caesarea. In each place he met with believers to say his farewells.

In Caesarea, a prophet named Agabus predicted the manner in which Paul would be bound in Jerusalem. The thought of Paul suffering agitated his friends, who urged him to change his plans. But Paul held firm. In a healthy life, we do not seek out suffering, but we do face suffering. In Paul's case, he was confident there was greater meaning in what he was about to endure.

While Paul was firm in his purpose, he sought out care and community at every stage of his journey. On one level, this was practical—he had to stay somewhere while the ship's workers unloaded cargo for seven days. On another level, though, it was intentional connection and forms a reminder that we do not have to face hardship alone. Paul was surrounded by close friends and people who cared for him. His friends, knowing danger lay ahead, nevertheless stayed with him for the entire journey to Jerusalem. What a gift to journey with another person into and through a hard season. We improve each other's well-being when we open ourselves to companionship on the way.

HEALTH TIP

Whether the wound or illness we carry is physical, spiritual, emotional, or relational, a large part of healing is having a support system. Who are the people you can count on to remain at your side even when you tell the truth? How can you be that kind of person for someone else? Have a conversation with someone about the healing journey you're on and the goals still ahead of you.

— DAILY HEALTH JOURNAL —

Number of steps................................   O Add 3 servings of vegetables

O Add 2,000 steps   O Add 3 glasses of water

Under Arrest

ACTS 21:17-19, 27-35

*After greeting them, he related one by one the things that
God had done among the Gentiles through his ministry.*
—Acts 21:19

THE BELIEVERS IN JERUSALEM WELCOMED the traveling band warmly. Paul met with James, Jesus' brother who was now leader of the church in Jerusalem, and other leaders to share what God had done through Paul's ministry among the Gentiles.

Paul was in Jerusalem for more than a week before trouble stirred. Jews from outside Jerusalem, who had known and opposed Paul during his travels, energized a mob with false accusations. His attackers would have killed him had representatives of the Roman government not intervened to quell the chaos. The safest thing for Paul under the circumstances was to be arrested, and this is what happened.

The more we read of Paul's story the more we see that he did not avoid the hard stuff. He didn't try to find a ministry niche where he could be comfortable and safe. For Paul that would have meant turning away from what God asked him to do.

The truth is that hard stuff happens in all of our lives. Broken relationships. Bad news from the doctor. An accident that shatters our plans. The bottom dropping out of our careful financial strategy. Identity theft. But the even greater truth is that in any of those moments, we are not separated from God. We don't lose our worth in God's eyes because we suffer. We may even be surprised to find ourselves drawing closer to God in these times.

HEALTH TIP

Sometimes we think that steps toward health and well-being must be gigantic or else they don't matter. The opposite is true. Nurture your awareness of signs of life, whether visible externally to others or known internally only to you. Celebrate every sign of life and reminder of healing, no matter how small. Every glimpse of joy, every close moment with God, every small step toward your goal matters.

— DAILY HEALTH JOURNAL —

Number of steps ....   ○ Add 3 servings of vegetables

○ Add 2,000 steps   ○ Add 3 glasses of water

Sailing for Rome
ACTS 27:12-20

We were being pounded by the storm so violently that on the next day they began to throw the cargo overboard.
—Acts 27:18

PAUL'S ARREST LED TO A SERIES of confusing religious and civil trials and general conundrum about what could be done about this man who had not actually committed a crime but against whom the crowds were hostile. In every defense, Paul emphasized the resurrection of Jesus as the crucial point of Christian faith. After trials in Jerusalem, Paul was sent to the Roman governor in Caesarea, where he had a prolonged house arrest with no resolution of charges against him. Paul then invoked his rights as a Roman citizen for a trial in Rome.

Delays in travel meant that sailing became dangerous because of seasonal weather conditions. They would have to spend the winter somewhere—but where? The ship's authorities pressed on for a suitable harbor, but they lost their race against the sea and found themselves pounded by unrelenting stormy weather. "All hope of our being saved was at last abandoned," Luke tells us (Acts 27:20).

Could there be any more profound picture of hopelessness than being tossed on a violent sea out of range of any rescue operations and throwing provisions overboard in a last ditch effort for survival? This image raises the question of how we find hope in hopelessness. Remaining resilient in hopeless situations begins long before the trying circumstances arise. How would you evaluate your overall well-being? Are you building the habits and support networks that would allow you to see light in the darkest times?

HEALTH TIP

If you live in a place where the seasons change, chances are you have to adapt your exercise routine. Or the season of your life or work might change and call for a shift in routine. Avoid relying on one type of movement. Experiment with various activities that will serve you well in various seasons to keep you up and moving and on the path toward wholeness.

— DAILY HEALTH JOURNAL —

Number of steps................................   ⭕ Add 3 servings of vegetables
⭕ Add 2,000 steps   ⭕ Add 3 glasses of water

Run Aground

ACTS 27:39-44

But the centurion, wishing to save Paul, kept them from carrying out their plan. He ordered those who could swim to jump overboard first and make for the land.

—Acts 27:43

FOR TWO STORMY WEEKS, the ship Paul was aboard drifted across the Adriatic Sea. Paul, a prisoner whose own life was in danger because of decisions outside his control, was the source of hope on that ship. He stood up and spoke of hope and courage. He prodded everyone to eat and keep up their strength. He publicly gave thanks to God even in these circumstances.

Finally, land came within sight. The plan was to run the ship ashore. But it struck a reef, and the force of the waves was rapidly breaking the ship apart. The lives of prisoners, including Paul, were now further imperiled because of the risk that they might swim to freedom. Soldiers planned to simply kill the prisoners before this could happen. The centurion in charge, who himself would have to answer for the loss of the prisoners, put a stop to this idea. He had come to see Paul in a new light—someone who was a leader and an encourager.

Instead of killing the prisoners, the centurion ordered that anyone—prisoner or not—who was able to swim to shore should do so. The rest followed, kept afloat on debris from the broken ship. Everyone reached land safely.

In the moment, we may be tempted to make the desperate, self-protecting choice. Encouragement and hope may come from unexpected sources. Thinking about the wellness of others can play a significant role in our own health and well-being.

HEALTH TIP

As determined as we might be to make changes in our health habits, we all experience setbacks. "Two steps forward, one step back" is a reality in any dimension of life. But if we turn around and see where we have come from, we can see that the effort is indeed taking us where we want to go. Don't beat yourself up about a setback. Just start again and keep going.

– DAILY HEALTH JOURNAL –

Number of steps ....   O Add 3 servings of vegetables

O Add 2,000 steps   O Add 3 glasses of water

Island of Healing

ACTS 28:1, 7-10, 16

*After this happened, the rest of the people on the
island who had diseases also came and were cured.*

—Acts 28:9

SOON ENOUGH, THE BELEAGUERED sailors learned they had found refuge on Malta near the toe of Italy. Here they would spend the winter before continuing to Rome. Publius, the leading personality on the island, offered hospitality. When Publius was sick, Paul visited him and prayed for him. Seeing his ministry, others on the island who were sick also came to Paul for healing. Such a positive relationship developed that when it was time for Paul to sail on to Rome on another ship, residents of the island made sure Paul and his friends had all the provisions they needed.

This was not a ministry season that was planned. Paul did not decide to spend the winter on Malta. In fact, he had warned the ship's authority that they ought to find a harbor sooner, before the storm, rather than press on. Had they heeded his advice, they would not have been shipwrecked, and he would not have met Publius or any of the people on Malta. Whether planned or not, however, Paul met people in their need and offered something to make their lives better.

Paul shows us the beautiful potential that comes from circumstances we don't choose and the opportunities to offer healing hope to people we never expected to meet. As we wait out the winters of our lives—and they do come—we can welcome the opportunities to connect with others in unexpected ways.

HEALTH TIP

No one knows your body as well as you do. This is one reason why regular self-exams play an important role in physical health. Breast-exams for women and testicular exams for men should be done monthly to increase the chance that you'll detect a change while it is small. Early detection of cancer greatly increases the chances of recovery. Your doctor can help you learn how to perform these important self-exams.

— DAILY HEALTH JOURNAL —

Number of steps ....   O Add 3 servings of vegetables

O Add 2,000 steps   O Add 3 glasses of water

Rome in Sight

ACTS 28:16–24

After they had set a day to meet with him,
they came to him at his lodgings in great numbers.
—Acts 28:23

AFTER THREE MONTHS ON MALTA, Paul—still a prisoner—sailed for Rome on a ship that had also wintered on the island. In Rome, Paul lived in a rented house under guard, rather than in a rugged Roman prison. He was not accused of a dangerous crime and was not seriously considered a political threat, so he was free to host his friends and invite people in for conversations.

Though the journey to Rome was triggered by legal issues rather than missionary endeavor, Paul's priorities were still to preach good news about Jesus. In this circumstance, he was not free to seek out a Jewish synagogue as he had in so many other cities. Instead he invited Jewish leaders to the place where he stayed. As always, his presentation was based in the Hebrew Scriptures. And as always, some were convinced that Jesus was the Messiah who brought the kingdom of God while others refused to believe.

Paul had long thought of visiting Rome. In fact, he had already written the book of Romans, a letter to the Roman church, while he was in Corinth. Most likely he envisioned a missionary journey rather than life-threatening shipwreck and house arrest under constant guard. Whatever the circumstances, his ministry there was fruitful.

Opportunity to do God's work is everywhere. Wherever we find ourselves, and whatever circumstances bring us there, we can be secure that God is at work in and through us in ways that bring hope and healing to others.

HEALTH TIP

In an era of the Internet and social media, and even online dating, people build connections in all sorts of ways. These relationships can be genuine and profound—or they can make it easy for us to hide behind the image we would like people to have of us. Make sure that the relationships you spend your time in, regardless of their form, are ones that support your health goals and well-being.

— DAILY HEALTH JOURNAL —

Number of steps ....   O Add 3 servings of vegetables

O Add 2,000 steps   O Add 3 glasses of water

Proclaiming the Kingdom
ACTS 28:30-31

*He lived there two whole years at his own expense
and welcomed all who came to him.*
—Acts 28:30

EARLY CHRISTIAN TRADITION SUGGESTS that Paul was released after two years of house arrest and went on to minister in other places. The gospel has widened from its beginnings in Jerusalem to the most influential cities of the Roman Empire, including Rome itself.

Luke's account of the early church, especially the life of Paul, ends on a triumphant note. Luke chooses not to tell us the details of the disposition of Paul's legal case in Rome. Luke's purpose was not to tell the life of Paul but to recount the wide spread of the gospel, which he has done. His focus in writing is the same as Paul's focus in preaching—the kingdom of God.

The kingdom of God is a welcoming kingdom meant for all people to find healing and wholeness that God intends for them, so it is fitting that Luke ends his account with a picture of Paul welcoming all who came to him to hear about the kingdom of God.

In what ways has the message of God's kingdom reached into your life to bring healing and wholeness? In what ways might you carry that message in ever-widening circles to others who need the wholeness that comes by receiving God's love and care? As you consider the journey you have taken for the last six weeks as you've walked with Paul, think about the ways you can be a co-laborer in the gospel with Paul.

HEALTH TIP

Congratulations! You've come to the end of six weeks of *Walking with Paul.* You can look back on the journey and see both the triumphs and the obstacles. You can celebrate the results. You can look at the future and formulate your next goals. Now that you've come this far, where would you like to go? You can get there, a step at a time!

— DAILY HEALTH JOURNAL —

Number of steps............ ○ Add 3 servings of vegetables
○ Add 2,000 steps ○ Add 3 glasses of water

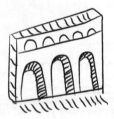

Week Six in Review

YOU'VE ACCOMPLISHED SOMETHING in the last six weeks! You've set goals and moved toward them. While there might have been setbacks, you've seen that God invites you to continue moving forward. You can give yourself the same grace and mercy you extend to others.

Where will you go from here? Now that you're in a rhythm of setting simple goals for changing your health habits and seeing steady results, consider what goals you might set for the next six weeks. Will you continue to add steps to your day? Find new forms of recreation to enjoy? Be intentional about spending time with friends who bring you encouragement and joy? Seek ways to fulfill a new calling in your life? Explore new spiritual practices? All these things contribute to your health and well-being. Use this jumping off point to make pursuing greater wellness a lifelong habit, one step at a time.

Transfer your daily steps in the space below. If you set a goal for all three categories, put checkmarks in the boxes where you reached your goal for each day.

Number of steps	Add 2,000 steps	Add 3 vegetables	Add 3 glasses of water
Day 1	O	O	O
Day 2	O	O	O
Day 3	O	O	O
Day 4	O	O	O
Day 5	O	O	O
Day 6	O	O	O
Day 7	O	O	O

— Congratulations! —

YOU HAVE COMPLETED *Walking with Paul.* By increasing your steps, adding 3 servings of vegetables, and adding 3 glasses of water each day, you have taken some steps in the right direction.

It's important to continue the lifestyle changes you've made during the last six weeks. Treat yourself to a new pair of walking shoes. Explore a museum, zoo, or nature preserve. You may even consider walking in a charity 5K with a friend. Think of fun ways to reward yourself that will relate to your new lifestyle and motivate you to continue your new habits.

Please take a few minutes to answer the following questions and return the completed form to your project coordinator.

Name: _____

Congregation or Community Organization: _____

_____

1. I was able to add 2,000 steps to my daily activity.
   ○ Never   ○ Seldom   ○ Sometimes   ○ Often   ○ Always

2. I was able to add 3 servings of vegetables to my daily meals.
   ○ Never   ○ Seldom   ○ Sometimes   ○ Often   ○ Always

3. I was able to add 3 glasses of water to my fluid fluids.
   ○ Never   ○ Seldom   ○ Sometimes   ○ Often   ○ Always

4. I found *Walking with Paul* to be helpful and it inspired me to reach my goals.
   ○ Never   ○ Seldom   ○ Sometimes   ○ Often   ○ Always

5. How many days a week do you engage in some type of mild to moderate physical activity (walking slowly, gardening, housework, window shopping, and so on)?   Days per week _____

6. How many days a week do you engage in some type of moderate to vigorous physical activity (brisk walking, running, riding a bike, dancing, playing a sport and so on)?   Days per week _____

CUT HERE

7. Which answer best describes how you feel about the following?

	I have no plans to	I plan to in the future	I plan to immediately	I have been doing so for *fewer* than six months	I have been doing so for *more* than six months
Increasing physical activity					
Improving nutrition					

8. To what degree do you feel that your physical health and spiritual health are connected?

○ Not at all   ○ Quite a bit

○ A little bit   ○ Extremely

○ Moderately

9. What comments would you like to share with the project coordinator?

*Thank you for participating! Please return this
form to the project coordinator in your
congregation or community organization.*

CUT HERE ↷

CONTINUE THE JOURNEY TO HEALTH

More from the Ways to Wellness series ...

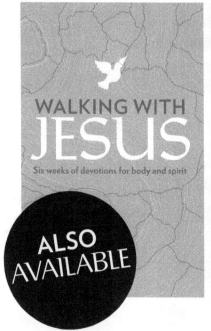

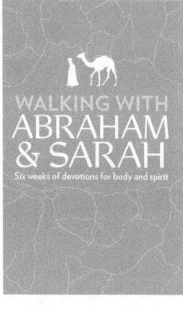

Work on health goals for six weeks while meditating on Scripture readings that follow the walking routes of **JESUS** and **ABRAHAM & SARAH**.

About the Author

SUSAN MARTINS MILLER has been a
writer and editor for over 30 years,
creating faith-based resources for
children and adults to use both at
home and in congregational settings. She
holds a master's degree in biblical studies
(New Testament) from Trinity Evangelical
Divinity School.

Walking with Paul is part of the Ways to
Wellness series, which also includes *Walking
with Jesus* and *Walking with Abraham and Sarah*.

Printed in the USA
CPSIA information can be obtained
at www.ICGtesting.com
LVHW090226270824
789263LV00002B/59

9 781621 440673